While every precaution has been taken in the preparation of this book, the publisher assumes no responsibility for errors or omissions, or for damages resulting from the use of the information contained herein.

WEIGHT GAIN SOLUTION YOUR COMPLETE GUIDE TO HEALTHY AND SUSTAINABLE WEIGHT GAIN

First edition. August 5, 2023.

Copyright © 2023 Ben S Roberts.

Written by Ben S Roberts.

<u>**Be empowered with comprehensive knowl-
edge and actionable strategies to reach your
weight gain goals, while prioritizing your
health.**</u>

Introduction

Welcome to "The Weight Gain Solution: Your Complete Guide to Healthy and Sustainable Weight Gain." This book is designed to empower you with comprehensive knowledge and actionable strategies to reach your weight gain goals while prioritizing your health. Whether you've struggled to gain weight in the past or you're looking to add muscle mass, this guide will provide you with the tools and guidance you need to achieve success.

Why You Need This Book

Weight gain is often overshadowed by the more common topic of weight loss, but it's equally important for those who are underweight or seeking to improve their physical performance. Many people face challenges in gaining weight due to various factors, such as a fast metabolism, busy lifestyles, or limited access to reliable information. This book aims to fill that knowledge gap and offer practical solutions for healthy weight gain.

By reading this book, you'll gain insights into the factors that influence weight gain, learn how to set achievable goals, and discover effective strategies to make progress in your weight gain journey. We believe that every individual has the potential to achieve their desired weight in a safe and sustainable way, and this book will be your guide on that path.

What to Expect

"The Weight Gain Solution" is organized in a logical and progressive manner to help you build a solid foundation of understanding and then move towards implementing practical steps for weight gain. The chapters are designed to cover various aspects of weight gain, including nutrition, exercise, and overcoming challenges along the way.

Each chapter contains valuable information backed by scientific research and real-world experience. You'll find useful tips, strategies, and even motivational anecdotes to keep you inspired throughout your journey. We want this book to be your go-to resource, answering your questions and guiding you through any obstacles you may encounter.

How to Use This Book

To make the most of this guide, we encourage you to read it sequentially from the beginning. This will help you grasp the fundamental concepts of weight gain before diving into more specific topics. However, feel free to skip ahead to a particular chapter if you're looking for targeted information on a particular aspect of weight gain.

In each chapter, you'll find actionable steps and practical advice that you can implement in your daily life. Take your time with the content and apply the tips at your own pace. Remember, this is not a crash diet or a quick-fix solution; it's a holistic approach to help you achieve sustainable weight gain while nurturing your overall well-being.

Are you ready to embark on your weight gain journey? Let's get started on building a stronger, healthier, and more confident you. Turn the page, and let "The Weight Gain Solution" be your guide to a successful and fulfilling transformation.

Chapter 1: Understanding Weight Gain

Weight gain is a complex process that occurs when the amount of energy consumed through food and drink exceeds the amount of energy expended through physical activity and bodily functions. This excess energy is then stored in the body as fat, leading to weight gain over time.

There are several factors that contribute to weight gain, including genetics, lifestyle, and environmental factors. Some people may have a genetic predisposition to gain weight more easily than others, but weight gain ultimately comes down to a simple equation of energy balance.

It's important to understand that weight gain is not solely determined by calorie intake and expenditure. The type of food consumed also plays a role. Highly processed and high-calorie foods, such as sugary drinks, fast food, and snacks, can contribute to weight gain more than nutrient-dense and lower-calorie foods.

Additionally, sedentary behaviors, such as sitting or lying down for long periods of time, can also contribute to weight gain. Lack of physical activity decreases the amount of energy expended, leading to an imbalance between calorie intake and expenditure.

Another factor that can contribute to weight gain is stress. When we experience stress, our bodies release hormones, such as cortisol, which can increase appetite and lead to overeating. Moreover, people often turn to comfort foods, which are

What is weight gain?

Weight gain refers to the process of increasing one's body weight by adding pounds or kilograms above an individual's optimal or healthy weight for their height, age, and gender. It occurs when there is an imbalance between the energy consumed through food and drinks and the energy expended through physical activity and bodily functions.

Weight gain can be a desired goal for individuals who are underweight or those looking to improve their overall health, enhance athletic performance, or achieve a more balanced physique. It is essential to approach weight gain in a balanced and sustainable manner, ensuring that the additional weight is primarily in the form of muscle rather than excess body fat.

For individuals aiming to gain weight in a healthy way, a combination of proper nutrition and exercise is essential. This involves strategically increasing caloric intake while prioritizing nutrient-dense foods rich in proteins, carbohydrates, healthy fats, vitamins, and minerals. Regular strength training exercises are crucial to stimulate muscle growth and promote healthy weight gain.

Gaining weight in a healthy manner not only involves consuming more calories but also making smart choices to ensure that the body receives all the essential nutrients it needs to support growth and repair. It is important to avoid relying solely on unhealthy, calorie-dense foods, as this can lead to an unhealthy increase in body fat and other potential health issues.

Why do some people have a hard time gaining weight?

I understand that weight gain challenges can be multifaceted and deeply personal for individuals. While some people may find it easy to gain weight, others may struggle despite their efforts. Several factors contribute to this difficulty in gaining weight, and it's essential to approach the topic with sensitivity and understanding. Here are some common reasons why some individuals have a hard time gaining weight:

1. Metabolism and Genetics:

One of the primary factors influencing weight gain is an individual's metabolism, which refers to how efficiently their body burns calories. Some people naturally have a faster metabolism, meaning they burn calories at a higher rate, making it more challenging for them to maintain a caloric surplus needed for weight gain. Additionally, genetics can play a role in determining body composition and distribution of fat and muscle.

2. High Energy Expenditure:

Individuals with an active lifestyle or physically demanding occupations may struggle to gain weight because they burn a significant amount of calories throughout the day. Athletes, for example, often have high energy expenditures due to intense training and exercise, which can offset the caloric surplus required for weight gain.

3. Low Appetite:

Some people have naturally lower appetites, which can make it challenging for them to consume the necessary amount of calories needed for weight gain. This might be influenced by factors such as stress, medical conditions, or certain medications that can suppress appetite.

4. Medical Conditions:

Underlying medical conditions can also hinder weight gain efforts. Conditions like hyperthyroidism, gastrointestinal disorders, or malabsorption issues may impact nutrient absorption, making it difficult for the body to retain essential calories and nutrients.

5. Psychological Factors:

Psychological factors can also play a significant role in weight gain challenges. Stress, anxiety, depression, or body image concerns can affect eating habits and overall well-being, potentially leading to difficulties in gaining weight.

6. Unhealthy Eating Habits:

While some individuals struggle to eat enough, others may find it challenging to make nutritious food choices. Relying on unhealthy, calorie-dense foods lacking essential nutrients can lead to weight gain in an unhealthy way, potentially causing other health issues.

7. Eating Disorders:

In severe cases, individuals struggling with eating disorders, such as anorexia nervosa or bulimia, face significant challenges in gaining weight. These disorders involve complex psychological and emotional factors that require professional intervention and support.

It's crucial to remember that every individual is unique, and the reasons behind weight gain challenges can vary widely. If you or someone you know is facing difficulties in gaining weight, seeking guidance from a healthcare professional, such as a registered dietitian or doctor, can provide personalized insights and support. A comprehensive evaluation can identify underlying issues and help develop a tailored plan to achieve healthy and sustainable weight gain while addressing any physical or psychological barriers.

The importance of healthy weight gain

Healthy weight gain is an essential aspect of overall well-being, especially for individuals who are underweight or have difficulty maintaining a healthy weight. While much attention is often given to weight loss, healthy weight gain is equally crucial for various reasons. Whether you're recovering from an illness, trying to build muscle, or simply aiming to reach a healthier weight, understanding the importance of healthy weight gain is vital.

1. Adequate Nutrition: Gaining weight in a healthy manner ensures that your body receives the necessary nutrients it

requires to function optimally. A well-balanced diet rich in proteins, carbohydrates, healthy fats, vitamins, and minerals helps support the body's growth, repair, and overall health. Avoiding crash diets and embracing nutrient-dense foods ensures that the weight gain is beneficial and sustainable in the long run.

2. Muscle and Bone Health: Healthy weight gain often involves building lean muscle mass, which contributes to better muscle strength, stability, and functionality. Regular strength training exercises promote bone health and reduce the risk of osteoporosis. Muscle mass also helps improve metabolism, making it easier to maintain a healthy weight and reduce the chances of chronic diseases such as diabetes and cardiovascular issues.

3. Boosting Energy Levels: Gaining weight in a healthy manner can increase energy levels, helping individuals feel more active and engaged in their daily activities. Proper weight gain can also alleviate fatigue and boost productivity, ultimately enhancing the quality of life.

4. Immune System Support: Adequate nutrition and a healthy weight play a significant role in bolstering the immune system. When the body receives the necessary nutrients to function optimally, it becomes more resilient to infections and diseases, leading to a reduced risk of illnesses.

5. Psychological Well-being: Being underweight can lead to feelings of insecurity, low self-esteem, and body image issues. Gaining weight in a healthy manner can boost self-confidence and overall mental well-being. It allows individuals to feel more comfortable in their bodies and fosters a positive relationship with food and exercise.

6. Hormonal Balance: Hormonal imbalances are common in individuals with insufficient body weight. Hormones play a

crucial role in regulating various bodily functions, and maintaining a healthy weight helps ensure hormonal balance. This can lead to improved mood, better sleep, and enhanced reproductive health.

7. Improved Cardiovascular Health: For some underweight individuals, gaining weight can be crucial in supporting cardiovascular health. Adequate body fat levels and a balanced diet can help maintain healthy cholesterol and blood pressure levels, reducing the risk of heart-related issues.

8. Faster Recovery: Individuals recovering from illness, surgery, or injury often require extra nutrients and energy to heal properly. Healthy weight gain during the recovery process aids in tissue repair, reduces healing time, and enhances overall recovery outcomes.

9. Prevention of Undernutrition: Chronic undernutrition can lead to various deficiencies and health complications. Healthy weight gain helps prevent the risks associated with nutrient deficiencies, promoting optimal health and reducing the likelihood of developing malnutrition-related conditions.

In conclusion, healthy weight gain is not only about achieving a desired physical appearance but also about promoting overall health and well-being. It is crucial to adopt a balanced approach to nutrition, exercise, and lifestyle choices when aiming for weight gain. If you are concerned about your weight or nutritional needs, consulting with a healthcare professional or a registered dietitian can provide personalized guidance and support to help you achieve your goals safely and effectively.

Chapter 2: Nutrition for Weight Gain

How many calories do you need?

To determine how many calories you need to gain weight in a healthy manner, you must consider your Total Daily Energy Expenditure (TDEE). TDEE represents the total number of calories your body burns in a day, including the calories required for basal metabolic rate (BMR), physical activity, and thermic effect of food (TEF). To gain weight, you need to consume more calories than your TDEE, creating a caloric surplus.

Calculating TDEE involves the following steps:

1. **Calculate Basal Metabolic Rate (BMR):** BMR represents the number of calories your body requires to maintain basic physiological functions at rest. There are various formulas to estimate BMR, such as the Harris-Benedict equation or the Mifflin-St. Jeor equation. These formulas take into account your age, gender, weight, and height.

2. **Factor in Physical Activity Level:** Your TDEE also depends on your physical activity level. If you have a sedentary lifestyle, you'll have a lower activity factor, while those who are more active, such as athletes or individuals with physically demanding jobs, will have a higher activity factor. Multiply your BMR by the appropriate activity factor to account for daily activity.

3. **Add a Caloric Surplus:** To gain weight in a healthy manner, aim for a caloric surplus of about 250-500 calories per day. This modest surplus allows for gradual weight gain, mostly in the form of lean muscle mass rather than excessive fat.

For example, if your calculated TDEE is 2,000 calories per day and you want to gain weight, you may aim to consume around 2,250-2,500 calories per day.

It's essential to remember that weight gain should be gradual and steady. Rapid weight gain, achieved through excessive overeating, can lead to unhealthy fat accumulation and other health issues. Focusing on nutrient-dense foods, such as lean proteins, whole grains, fruits, vegetables, and healthy fats, will ensure that you gain weight while nourishing your body with essential nutrients.

Working with a registered dietitian or nutritionist can be highly beneficial in determining your personalized caloric needs and creating a balanced meal plan to support your weight gain goals. They can also monitor your progress and adjust your dietary intake as needed to ensure a safe and sustainable weight gain journey.

The role of macronutrients in weight gain

The role of macronutrients (carbohydrates, proteins, and fats) in weight gain is essential, as each macronutrient plays a specific role in the process of increasing body mass. Balancing these nutrients appropriately is crucial for healthy and effective weight gain.

1. Carbohydrates:

Carbohydrates are the body's primary source of energy. When you consume carbohydrates, they are broken down into glucose, which is then used to fuel various bodily functions, including physical activity and brain function. For weight gain, carbohydrates play a critical role in providing the energy needed to support workouts and increase overall daily caloric intake.

Complex Carbohydrates: Foods like whole grains (brown rice, quinoa, oats), fruits, vegetables, and legumes provide a steady release of glucose into the bloodstream. These complex carbohydrates help maintain energy levels and prevent blood sugar spikes and crashes.

Simple Carbohydrates: Foods like sugars and refined carbohydrates (sweets, sugary beverages, white bread) provide a quick source of energy but lack essential nutrients. Consuming too many simple carbohydrates can lead to unhealthy weight gain and potential health issues.

2. Proteins:

Proteins are vital for muscle repair, growth, and maintenance. When you engage in strength training or resistance exercises, small muscle tears occur. Protein is essential for repairing these muscle fibers, leading to muscle growth over time. Adequate protein intake is crucial for supporting muscle development during weight gain.

High-Quality Protein Sources: Foods like lean meats (chicken, turkey, lean beef), fish, eggs, dairy products, legumes, nuts, and plant-based proteins (tofu, tempeh, quinoa) provide essential amino acids necessary for muscle building and recovery.

3. Fats:

Fats are an essential part of a balanced diet and play several roles in weight gain. They are a concentrated source of energy, providing more calories per gram compared to carbohydrates and proteins. Healthy fats also support hormone production, nutrient absorption (fat-soluble vitamins), and overall cell function.

Healthy Fat Sources: Foods like avocados, nuts, seeds, olive oil, fatty fish (salmon, mackerel, sardines), and nut butters offer essential fatty acids and other beneficial nutrients.

Achieving Balance:

To promote healthy weight gain, it's essential to strike a balance between these macronutrients. While all macronutrients contribute to weight gain, it's crucial to prioritize nutrient-dense foods. A balanced diet that includes a mix of complex carbohydrates, high-quality proteins, and healthy fats provides the energy and nutrients necessary for supporting muscle growth and overall health.

Choosing nutrient-dense foods

Choosing nutrient-dense foods is crucial for achieving healthy weight gain while supporting overall well-being. Nutrient-dense foods provide a high concentration of essential vitamins, minerals, and other nutrients relative to their caloric content. Incorporating these foods into your diet ensures that you gain weight in a nourishing and balanced manner. Here are some tips for choosing nutrient-dense foods:

1. Emphasize Fruits and Vegetables:

Fruits and vegetables are rich sources of vitamins, minerals, fiber, and antioxidants. Include a variety of colorful fruits and vegetables in your diet to ensure you're getting a wide range of nutrients. Leafy greens, berries, citrus fruits, and cruciferous vegetables are particularly nutrient-dense options.

2. Opt for Whole Grains:

Whole grains, such as brown rice, quinoa, oats, and whole wheat, are more nutrient-dense than refined grains. They provide essential nutrients like fiber, B-vitamins, and minerals. Whole grains can also help regulate blood sugar levels and promote satiety.

3. Choose Lean Proteins:

Lean proteins are excellent choices for weight gain as they provide essential amino acids for muscle growth and repair. Opt for lean meats like skinless chicken, turkey, lean beef, or pork. Fish, eggs, dairy products, legumes, and plant-based protein sources like tofu and tempeh are also valuable options.

4. Include Healthy Fats:

Healthy fats are an important component of a nutrient-dense diet. Foods like avocados, nuts, seeds, olive oil, and fatty fish provide essential fatty acids and fat-soluble vitamins. Use these fats in moderation to add flavor and nutrition to your meals.

5. Incorporate Dairy or Dairy Alternatives:

Dairy products, like Greek yogurt and cottage cheese, are nutrient-dense sources of protein, calcium, and other essential nutrients. If you follow a plant-based diet or have lactose intolerance, choose fortified dairy alternatives like almond milk, soy milk, or oat milk to ensure you're getting similar nutrients.

6. Include Nuts and Seeds:

Nuts and seeds are calorie-dense and provide healthy fats, protein, fiber, vitamins, and minerals. They can be excellent snacks or additions to meals and smoothies.

7. Avoid Empty-Calorie Foods:

Minimize or avoid foods with empty calories, such as sugary snacks, sugary beverages, and processed foods high in added sugars and unhealthy fats. These foods can lead to unhealthy weight gain without providing valuable nutrients.

8. Read Nutrition Labels:

When shopping for packaged foods, read the nutrition labels to identify nutrient-dense choices. Look for products that are low in added sugars, sodium, and unhealthy fats while providing essential nutrients.

9. Plan Balanced Meals:

Aim to create balanced meals that include a mix of macronutrients and various food groups. This ensures that you get a wide range of nutrients to support your weight gain goals and overall health.

By incorporating nutrient-dense foods into your diet, you'll support your weight gain journey while nourishing your body with essential nutrients. Working with a registered dietitian can be beneficial in creating a personalized meal plan that meets your specific needs and preferences while promoting healthy weight gain.

Meal planning for weight gain

Choosing nutrient-dense foods is crucial for achieving healthy weight gain while supporting overall well-being. Nutrient-dense foods provide a high concentration of essential vitamins, minerals, and other nutrients relative to their caloric content. Incorporating these foods into your diet ensures that you gain weight in a nourishing and balanced mannern

Eating more frequently and smart snacking

Eating more frequently and incorporating smart snacking into your daily routine can be beneficial strategies for healthy weight gain. These practices help ensure a steady supply of nutrients and calories throughout the day, support muscle growth, and prevent excessive hunger that may lead to unhealthy food choices. Here's how you can optimize your eating frequency and snacking habits for a successful weight gain journey:

1. Frequent, Balanced Meals:

Instead of sticking to the traditional three meals per day, consider dividing your daily caloric intake into five to six smaller meals. Eating every 3-4 hours helps maintain a consistent flow of nutrients, supports energy levels, and prevents prolonged periods of hunger. Each meal should consist of a balance of macronutrients - protein, carbohydrates, and healthy fats - to provide sustained energy and promote muscle growth.

2. Don't Skip Breakfast:

Breakfast is a crucial meal, especially when trying to gain weight. Starting your day with a nutrient-dense breakfast sets a positive tone for the rest of the day. Include a mix of protein, whole grains, and fruits to provide essential nutrients and energy to kickstart your metabolism.

3. Pre- and Post-Workout Nutrition:

If you engage in regular physical activity, pay attention to your pre- and post-workout nutrition. Consume a small, easily digestible snack containing carbohydrates and protein before your workout to fuel your exercise session. Afterward, have a protein-rich snack to aid in muscle recovery and growth.

4. Smart Snacking:

Snacking can be an effective way to boost caloric intake and provide extra nutrients between meals. However, make smart choices by opting for nutrient-dense snacks rather than empty-calorie treats. Choose snacks that combine protein, healthy fats, and carbohydrates for a well-rounded option.

5. Nutrient-Dense Snack Options:

- **Greek yogurt with berries and a drizzle of honey**
- **Whole-grain crackers with hummus**
- **Mixed nuts and dried fruits**
- **Apple slices with nut butter**
- **Cottage cheese with sliced peaches**
- **Avocado on whole-grain toast**
- **Trail mix with nuts and seeds**

6. Portion Control:

While snacking can be beneficial for weight gain, it's essential to control portion sizes. Overeating, even with nutrient-dense snacks, can lead to excessive weight gain, including unhealthy fat accumulation.

7. Listen to Your Hunger and Fullness Cues:

Pay close attention to your body's indications of hunger and fullness. Don't force yourself to eat when you're not hungry, but aim to eat before you become overly hungry. Staying in tune with your body's cues helps maintain a healthy relationship with food.

8. Stay Hydrated:

Proper hydration is crucial for overall health and digestion. However, avoid drinking large amounts of fluids right before or during meals, as it can cause early satiety. Drink water between meals to avoid diluting your appetite.

9. Be Consistent:

Consistency is key to successful weight gain. Make eating more frequently and smart snacking a routine part of your daily life. Stick to your meal and snack schedule as closely as possible.

10. Monitor Progress:

Keep track of your weight gain progress and how you feel throughout the day. Adjust your meal frequency and snack choices based on your body's response and feedback.

By eating more frequently and choosing nutrient-dense snacks, you can ensure a steady intake of essential nutrients, support muscle growth, and maintain a positive relationship with food. Pair these practices with a well-balanced diet and regular exercise, and you'll be on your way to achieving healthy and sustainable weight gain.

Chapter 3: Supplementing for Weight Gain

- What supplements are helpful for weight gain?

While it's essential to primarily focus on a well-balanced diet and strength training to achieve healthy weight gain, some supplements can support your efforts. It's crucial to remember that supplements should not replace a nutritious diet but rather complement it. Always consult with a healthcare professional or a registered dietitian before starting any new supplements, as individual needs may vary. Here are some supplements that may be helpful for weight gain:

Supplemental protein: Protein is essential for building and repairing muscle. Protein supplements like whey protein, casein protein, or plant-based protein powders can be useful for individuals who struggle to consume enough protein through whole foods. These supplements can be convenient and help meet your protein needs, especially after workouts.

Creatine: Creatine is a naturally occurring compound that plays a significant role in energy production during high-intensity exercise. It has been shown to increase muscle mass and strength when combined with resistance training. For those looking to build muscle, creatine supplementation may provide some benefits.

Weight Gainers: Weight gainer supplements typically contain a mix of carbohydrates, protein, and fats to provide a high-calorie boost. They can be useful for individuals who struggle to consume enough calories from regular food sources. However, be mindful of added sugars and choose products with quality ingredients.

Omega-3 Fatty Acids: Omega-3 fatty acids are essential fats that offer numerous health benefits. While they may not directly contribute to weight gain, they support overall health, reduce inflammation, and enhance recovery, which can indirectly support your weight gain goals.

Branched-Chain Amino Acids (BCAAs): BCAAs are a group of essential amino acids that play a crucial role in muscle protein synthesis. They can aid in muscle recovery and reduce muscle breakdown during exercise, potentially supporting muscle gain.

Vitamin and Mineral Supplements: Ensuring adequate intake of vitamins and minerals is vital for overall health. A multivitamin or specific supplement for any deficiencies can be helpful, especially if you have dietary restrictions or specific nutrient needs.

Probiotics: A healthy gut is essential for optimal nutrient absorption and overall well-being. Probiotic supplements can support gut health, which may indirectly impact weight gain by improving nutrient absorption.

Healthy Fats: Incorporating healthy fats from sources like fish oil or flaxseed oil can help increase calorie intake and support overall health.

Healthy fats, also known as monounsaturated and polyunsaturated fats, are essential components of a well-balanced diet. Unlike saturated and trans fats, which are considered less healthy and should be limited, healthy fats offer numerous health benefits and play a crucial role in maintaining overall well-being. Here's more information about healthy fats:

1. Types of Healthy Fats: a. Monounsaturated Fats: These fats are found in high amounts in foods such as olive oil, avocados, nuts (e.g., almonds, cashews, peanuts), and seeds (e.g., sunflower seeds, pumpkin seeds). They have been associated with reducing bad cholesterol levels (LDL) and lowering the risk of heart disease.

b. Polyunsaturated Fats: This category includes two primary types of essential fats:

- Omega-3 Fatty Acids: Found in fatty fish (e.g., salmon, mackerel, sardines), flaxseeds, chia seeds, walnuts, and some fortified foods. Omega-3s are well-known for their anti-inflammatory properties and their role in supporting heart and brain health.
- Omega-6 Fatty Acids: Found in vegetable oils (e.g., soybean oil, corn oil, sunflower oil), nuts, and seeds. While omega-6 fats are essential, a balanced intake of omega-3 and omega-6 is crucial for maintaining a healthy ratio between the two.

Health Benefits of Healthy Fats:

- Heart Health: Monounsaturated and polyunsaturated fats have been associated with reducing bad cholesterol levels (LDL) and triglycerides, which are risk factors for heart disease. They can also increase good cholesterol levels (HDL) that help protect the heart.
- Brain Function: Omega-3 fatty acids, in particular, are essential for brain health and cognitive function. They play a role in

maintaining the structure of brain cells and are involved in neurotransmitter function.

- Inflammation: Healthy fats, especially omega-3 fatty acids, have anti-inflammatory properties that can help reduce inflammation in the body. Chronic inflammation is linked to various chronic diseases.
- Skin Health: Healthy fats contribute to skin health and can help maintain a smooth and supple complexion. They also play a role in reducing skin dryness and irritation.
- Nutrient Absorption: Fat is necessary for the absorption of fat-soluble vitamins (A, D, E, and K) in the body. Consuming healthy fats alongside nutrient-rich foods enhances the absorption of these essential vitamins.

1. Daily Intake and Moderation: While healthy fats offer numerous benefits, they are calorie-dense, containing nine calories per gram. Therefore, portion control is essential, especially if you're aiming to gain weight healthily. Replacing unhealthy fats (saturated and trans fats) with healthy fats is a practical approach to improving overall health.
2. Cooking with Healthy Fats: When cooking, opt for healthier cooking oils like olive oil, canola oil, or avocado oil instead of solid fats like butter or lard. These oils are better for heart health and provide a source of healthy fats.

Incorporating healthy fats into your diet can be beneficial for various aspects of your health, including heart health, brain function, and skin health. Remember to enjoy these fats in moderation and alongside a balanced diet rich in fruits, vegetables, whole grains, and lean proteins for overall well-being.

The pros and cons of weight gain supplements

Weight gain supplements can be a controversial topic, as they are designed to help individuals increase their caloric intake and gain weight. While some people may find them beneficial in certain situations, it's essential to consider both the pros and cons before deciding to use weight gain supplements.

Pros of Weight Gain Supplements:

1. Convenient Calorie Boost: Weight gain supplements typically come in powdered or liquid forms that can be easily mixed with water, milk, or other beverages. They provide a quick and convenient way to increase calorie intake, especially for individuals who struggle to eat large quantities of food.
2. Nutrient Fortification: Some weight gain supplements are fortified with essential vitamins, minerals, and macronutrients, offering a comprehensive nutritional profile. This can be beneficial for those with dietary restrictions or who have difficulty consuming a well-rounded diet.
3. Muscle Support: Many weight gain supplements contain protein, which is essential for muscle repair and growth. For individuals looking to build muscle mass, these supplements can be a helpful addition to their diet and exercise routine.
4. Faster Recovery: Weight gain supplements with added protein and carbohydrates can aid in post-workout recovery by replenishing glycogen stores and providing essential nutrients to support muscle repair.

Cons of Weight Gain Supplements:

1. High in Added Sugars and Artificial Ingredients: Some weight gain supplements may be high in added sugars and artificial

ingredients, which can negatively impact overall health. Excessive sugar consumption can lead to weight gain in the form of fat rather than muscle.

2. Unbalanced Nutrition: Relying too heavily on weight gain supplements may lead to an imbalanced diet, with an overemphasis on certain nutrients and a lack of variety from whole foods.

3. Digestive Issues: Some people may experience digestive discomfort, bloating, or other gastrointestinal issues when consuming weight gain supplements, particularly if they contain certain additives or ingredients that don't agree with their system.

4. Cost: Weight gain supplements can be expensive, especially if used regularly. This cost may not be sustainable for some individuals in the long run.

5. Not a Substitute for Real Food: Weight gain supplements should never replace real, nutrient-dense foods. While they can be a helpful addition to a balanced diet, whole foods provide a wide array of nutrients that supplements cannot fully replicate.

6. Weight Gain vs. Fat Gain: It's essential to be mindful of the type of weight being gained when using supplements. Excessive consumption of high-calorie supplements without an appropriate exercise routine may lead to an unhealthy increase in body fat rather than lean muscle mass.

In conclusion, weight gain supplements can be a useful tool for certain individuals, such as athletes, bodybuilders, or those with specific dietary needs. However, they should not be relied upon as the primary means of weight gain. It's crucial to use them in moderation, alongside a well-balanced diet, and under the guidance of a healthcare professional or a registered dietitian. Whenever possible, focus on obtaining essential nutrients from whole, nutrient-dense foods to support overall health and well-being.

Choosing the right supplements for your needs

Choosing the right supplements for your needs requires careful consideration and an understanding of your individual health goals and requirements. Here are some steps to help you make informed decisions:

1. Assess Your Nutritional Needs: Before selecting any supplements, evaluate your diet and lifestyle to identify potential nutrient gaps or deficiencies. Consider factors such as age, gender, activity level, dietary restrictions, and any health conditions you may have. A healthcare professional or a registered dietitian can conduct a comprehensive assessment and guide you in determining specific nutrient needs.

2. Prioritize Whole Foods: Supplements should not be a replacement for a balanced diet. Focus on obtaining nutrients from whole, nutrient-dense foods whenever possible. Aim to consume a variety of fruits, vegetables, whole grains, lean proteins, and healthy fats to meet your nutritional requirements.

3. Identify Targeted Goals: Determine your specific health and fitness goals. Whether it's improving cardiovascular health, building muscle, supporting bone health, or boosting immunity, knowing your objectives will help you choose supplements that align with those goals.

4. Research and Read Labels: Be an informed consumer and research the supplements you are considering. Look for reputable brands that have undergone third-party testing for quality and safety. Read product labels to understand the

ingredients, dosages, and any potential allergens or additives.

5. Consider Individual Nutrients: If you have identified specific nutrient deficiencies or needs, consider individual supplements that address those concerns. For example, if you are low in vitamin D, a vitamin D supplement might be appropriate. Always choose supplements that match your unique requirements.

6. Look for Synergistic Formulations: Some supplements come in combinations that provide complementary nutrients, enhancing their effectiveness. For instance, a calcium and vitamin D combination may benefit bone health.

7. Understand Dosages: Pay attention to recommended dosages and follow the guidelines provided by the supplement manufacturer or your healthcare professional. Avoid megadosing, as excessive intake of certain nutrients can be harmful.

8. Check for Interactions: If you are taking medications or have existing health conditions, consult with a healthcare professional to ensure that the supplements you plan to take do not interact negatively with your medications or health status.

9. Consider Your Budget: Supplements can vary significantly in price. While quality is essential, consider your budget when selecting supplements. Focus on essential nutrients first before considering additional supplements.

10. Monitor and Adjust: After starting any new supplements, monitor their effects on your health and well-being. If you experience any adverse effects or if your needs change over time, be open to adjusting your supplement regimen accordingly.

Remember that each individual's nutritional needs are unique, and what works for one person may not be suitable for another. Consulting with a healthcare professional or a registered dietitian is the best way to ensure you are choosing the right supplements for your specific needs and goals. They can provide personalized guidance, recommend appropriate supplements, and help you achieve optimal health and well-being.

Supplement safety and best practices

Supplement safety is of utmost importance to ensure that you are getting the intended benefits without any adverse effects. Here are some best practices to follow when using supplements:

1. Consult with a Healthcare Professional: Before starting any new supplement, talk to your doctor or a registered dietitian, especially if you have underlying health conditions, are pregnant or breastfeeding, or are taking medications. They can provide personalized advice based on your health status and help you make informed decisions.

2. Choose Reputable Brands: Select supplements from reputable brands that follow Good Manufacturing Practices (GMP) and have undergone third-party testing for quality and safety. Look for certifications from organizations like USP, NSF International, or ConsumerLab, which verify the authenticity and purity of supplements.

3. Read Product Labels: Carefully read supplement labels to understand the ingredients, dosage, and any potential allergens. Avoid supplements with unnecessary fillers, artificial colors, or other additives that may not contribute to your health goals.

4. Stick to Recommended Dosages: Take supplements as directed on the label or as advised by your healthcare professional. Avoid exceeding the recommended dosages, as megadosing can lead to adverse effects and potential health risks.

5. Avoid Mixing Multiple Supplements Without Guidance: Be cautious when combining multiple supplements, as some nutrients can interact with each other or with medications. Seek

guidance from a healthcare professional to ensure safe combinations.

6. Report Adverse Effects: If you experience any unusual or negative reactions after taking a supplement, stop using it immediately and consult with your healthcare provider. They can help determine whether the supplement is causing the adverse effects and advise on the next steps.

7. Be Patient and Consistent: Supplements may take time to show noticeable effects. Stay patient and consistent with your supplement regimen, and remember that they are meant to complement a healthy lifestyle, including a balanced diet and regular exercise.

8. Store Properly: Store supplements in a cool, dry place, away from direct sunlight and out of reach of children and pets. Follow any storage instructions provided on the supplement packaging.

9. Consider Nutrient Interactions: Be aware of potential interactions between supplements and medications or other supplements. For instance, calcium may interfere with the absorption of certain medications, while vitamin K can interact with blood-thinning medications.

10. Avoid Buying Counterfeit or Expired Products: Purchase supplements from reliable sources and avoid buying counterfeit products or supplements past their expiration dates.

Remember that supplements should not replace a well-balanced diet. They are meant to complement your nutritional intake, address specific deficiencies or health concerns, and support your overall well-being. Proper research, consultation with a healthcare professional, and following best practices will help ensure that you are using supplements safely and effectively.

Chapter 4: Exercise for Weight Gain

Exercise plays a crucial role in weight gain, especially when the goal is to gain lean muscle mass and improve overall body composition. Here are some key points to consider when using exercise for weight gain:

1. Resistance Training: Resistance training, also known as strength training or weightlifting, is the most effective form of exercise for promoting muscle growth and weight gain. It involves using resistance, such as free weights, machines, or bodyweight, to challenge and stimulate the muscles. Focus on compound exercises that target multiple muscle groups, such as squats, deadlifts, bench presses, and pull-ups.

2. Progressive Overload: To stimulate muscle growth and weight gain, it's essential to apply the principle of progressive overload. Gradually increase the intensity of your workouts over time by adding more weight, increasing the number of repetitions, or changing the exercise variations. This progressive approach ensures continuous muscle adaptation and growth.

3. Volume and Frequency: Aim for a sufficient training volume, which is the total amount of work performed in a workout. This can be achieved by doing multiple sets and repetitions of each exercise. A frequency of 3 to 4 strength training sessions per week is generally effective for promoting muscle gain.

4. Compound Movements: Compound exercises engage multiple muscle groups simultaneously, making them more efficient for muscle growth compared to isolation exercises. Compound movements require more energy and promote the release of anabolic hormones, such as testosterone and growth hormone, which support muscle development.

5. Rest and Recovery: Adequate rest and recovery are essential for

muscle repair and growth. Allow each muscle group at least 48 hours of rest before training them again. During rest periods, muscles repair and become stronger, contributing to overall weight gain.

6. Nutrition: Exercise for weight gain should be complemented by a balanced and calorie-dense diet. Ensure you're consuming enough calories to support both your daily activities and your exercise routine. Include ample protein to provide the building blocks for muscle repair and growth.

7. Post-Workout Nutrition: Proper post-workout nutrition is essential for recovery and muscle growth. Consume a combination of carbohydrates and protein shortly after your workout to replenish glycogen stores and provide amino acids for muscle repair.

8. Stay Hydrated: Hydration is crucial for overall health and optimal exercise performance. Drink plenty of water throughout the day, including before, during, and after your workouts.

9. Track Progress: Keep track of your exercise routine, including the exercises performed, sets, repetitions, and weights used. Tracking your progress helps you identify improvements and adjust your workout plan accordingly.

10. Be Patient and Consistent: Building muscle and gaining weight takes time and dedication. Stay patient with your progress and remain consistent with your exercise routine and nutrition.

It's important to note that weight gain should be approached in a healthy and balanced manner. Avoid excessive calorie intake or over-training, as this can lead to unhealthy weight gain or increase the risk of injury. If you are new to strength training or have any health concerns, consider working with a certified personal trainer to create a safe and effective workout plan tailored to your needs and goals.

How much exercise do you need?

The amount of exercise needed to gain weight varies depending on individual factors such as metabolism, body composition, fitness level, and specific weight gain goals. However, the focus should be on exercises that promote muscle growth and strength. Here are some general guidelines:

1. Strength Training: For weight gain, prioritize strength training or resistance exercises. Aim for 3 to 4 strength training sessions per week. Each session should target different muscle groups to allow sufficient rest and recovery.

2. Exercise Duration: Aim for 45 minutes to 1 hour per strength training session. Spending more time on targeted exercises allows for sufficient volume and muscle stimulation.

3. Exercise Intensity: Use moderate to heavy weights that challenge your muscles. The number of repetitions and sets will depend on your specific program, but typically 3 to 5 sets of 6 to 12 repetitions per exercise is common.

4. Compound Movements: Include compound exercises like squats, deadlifts, bench presses, overhead presses, rows, and pull-ups. These movements engage multiple muscle groups and are effective for promoting muscle growth.

5. Cardiovascular Exercise: While cardiovascular exercise is important for overall health, limit its duration and intensity if the primary goal is weight gain. Focus more on strength training to avoid excessive calorie expenditure from cardio.

6. Rest and Recovery: Allow each muscle group at least 48 hours of rest before training them again. Rest and recovery are crucial for muscle repair and growth.

7. Progressive Overload: Continuously challenge your muscles by increasing the weight, repetitions, or sets over time. Progressive overload stimulates muscle growth and prevents plateaus.

8. Proper Nutrition: Alongside exercise, ensure you are consuming enough calories to support weight gain. A calorie surplus is necessary to promote weight gain, so focus on a balanced diet that includes an adequate amount of protein, carbohydrates, and healthy fats.

9. Stay Consistent: Consistency is key to seeing progress. Stick to your exercise routine and nutritional plan, and be patient as gaining weight, especially in the form of muscle, takes time.

10. Listen to Your Body: Pay attention to how your body responds to exercise and adjust your routine as needed. If you experience excessive fatigue or prolonged soreness, consider adding more rest days or reducing the intensity of your workouts.

Remember that individual responses to exercise can vary, and there is no one-size-fits-all approach to weight gain. It's essential to find a workout routine that suits your specific needs, preferences, and fitness level. If you're unsure about how to design an effective exercise plan for weight gain, consider seeking guidance from a certified personal trainer. They can assess your current fitness level, discuss your goals, and create a personalized workout program that aligns with your objectives. Working with a professional trainer can provide valuable support, motivation, and ensure you exercise safely and effectively to achieve your weight gain goals.

The relationship between exercise and weight gain

The positive relationship between exercise and weight gain is often misunderstood, as many people associate exercise with weight loss rather than weight gain. However, exercise can play a significant role in promoting healthy weight gain, especially when combined with proper nutrition and strength training. Here are some ways in which exercise can contribute to weight gain in a positive manner:

1. Muscle Growth: One of the primary benefits of exercise, especially strength training, is the stimulation of muscle growth. Resistance exercises cause microscopic tears in muscle fibers, and during the recovery phase, the muscles repair and grow stronger and larger. This increase in lean muscle mass contributes to weight gain in a healthy way.

2. Calorie Surplus: To gain weight, you need to consume more calories than your body burns. Exercise can help create a calorie surplus, as it increases your energy expenditure, allowing you to consume more calories to support muscle growth and weight gain.

3. Appetite Stimulation: Regular exercise can stimulate your appetite, making it easier to consume more calories. This can be especially beneficial for individuals who have a naturally low appetite or struggle to eat enough to support weight gain.

4. Improved Nutrient Absorption: Exercise enhances blood flow to the digestive system, which can improve nutrient absorption. This means that your body can better utilize the nutrients from the food you eat, supporting overall health and weight gain.

5. Bone Health: Weight-bearing exercises, such as strength training, can improve bone density and reduce the risk of osteoporosis. This is particularly important for individuals who are underweight or at risk of bone-related issues.

6. Metabolic Benefits: Regular exercise can boost your metabolism, even at rest. As you gain muscle mass, your body becomes more metabolically active, leading to increased calorie burning throughout the day.

7. Positive Body Composition: Exercise can help improve body composition by increasing muscle mass while reducing body fat percentage. This results in a healthier weight gain, with a focus on lean tissue rather than excess fat.

8. Mental Health: Regular exercise has numerous mental health

benefits, reducing stress, anxiety, and depression. Improved mental well-being can positively influence your appetite, eating habits, and overall motivation to pursue a healthy weight gain journey.

It's important to note that exercise alone may not lead to significant weight gain, especially if your calorie intake remains insufficient. Combining exercise with a well-balanced diet that provides adequate calories and nutrients is crucial for effective weight gain. Additionally, individual responses to exercise can vary, so it's essential to find an exercise routine that suits your preferences, fitness level, and weight gain goals.

Strength training and muscle-building exercises

Strength training and muscle-building exercises are not exclusive to men; they are equally beneficial and important for women. Strength training helps women build muscle, improve bone density, boost metabolism, and enhance overall fitness and health. Here are some effective strength training exercises for women:

1. Squats: Squats are a fundamental lower body exercise that targets the quadriceps, hamstrings, glutes, and core. They can be performed with body weight, dumbbells, or a barbell.
2. Lunges: Lunges work the quadriceps, hamstrings, glutes, and calves. They can be done using body weight or with added resistance from dumbbells or a barbell.
3. Deadlifts: Deadlifts are excellent for targeting the hamstrings, glutes, lower back, and grip strength. They can be performed using a barbell, dumbbells, or kettlebells.
4. Bench Press: The bench press is an effective upper body exercise that targets the chest, shoulders, and triceps. It can be done with a barbell or dumbbells.
5. Shoulder Press: The shoulder press targets the deltoid muscles

and the triceps. It can be performed with dumbbells or a barbell.

6. Bent-Over Rows: Bent-over rows are great for working the upper back, lats, and biceps. They can be done with dumbbells or a barbell.

7. Push-Ups: Push-ups are a bodyweight exercise that targets the chest, shoulders, triceps, and core.

8. Pull-Ups/Chin-Ups: Pull-ups and chin-ups are challenging bodyweight exercises that target the back, biceps, and shoulders.

9. Hip Thrusts: Hip thrusts are excellent for targeting the glutes and hamstrings. They can be performed with body weight or using a barbell.

10. Dips: Dips target the triceps, chest, and shoulders. They can be done using parallel bars or assisted dip machines.

When performing strength training exercises, it's essential to use proper form and start with appropriate weights for your fitness level. Gradually increase the intensity and weight as you become more comfortable with the movements. Aim for 3 to 4 strength training sessions per week, with rest days in between to allow for muscle recovery and growth.

Strength training can be adapted to suit individual fitness goals and preferences. Women can use various training modalities, such as free weights, resistance bands, machines, or bodyweight exercises. Additionally, incorporating a variety of exercises into your routine can help target different muscle groups and provide a well-rounded workout.

· · · ·

Balancing cardio and resistance training for weight gain

Balancing cardio and resistance training is essential for weight gain in a healthy and effective way. While resistance training primarily focuses on building muscle mass, cardiovascular exercise offers several benefits for overall health and fitness. Here are some tips for balancing these two types of exercises to support weight gain:

1. Prioritize Resistance Training: When aiming to gain weight and build muscle, prioritize resistance training over cardio. Strength training is the most effective way to stimulate muscle growth, which contributes to weight gain in the form of lean body mass.

2. Frequency of Strength Training: Aim for 3 to 4 strength training sessions per week. Each session should target different muscle groups to allow sufficient rest and recovery.

3. Cardio Duration: Limit the duration of cardiovascular exercise to avoid excessive calorie expenditure. For weight gain, consider shorter and less frequent cardio sessions compared to those focused on weight loss or cardiovascular endurance.

4. Choose Low-Intensity Cardio: Opt for low-intensity cardio activities, such as walking, gentle cycling, or swimming. These activities help improve cardiovascular health without burning too many calories, allowing you to maintain a calorie surplus for weight gain.

5. Separate Cardio and Strength Training Sessions: If possible, perform cardio and resistance training on separate days. This allows you to focus on each type of exercise without compromising the intensity of either.

6. Timing of Cardio: If you prefer to do cardio on the same day as strength training, try to do it after your weightlifting session. This ensures that your energy and glycogen stores are not

depleted before your resistance training.

7. Adequate Nutrition: Ensure you consume enough calories to support both your exercise routine and weight gain goals. Proper nutrition is crucial for building muscle and supporting your energy needs.

8. Monitor Progress: Regularly assess your progress to ensure that your exercise routine is helping you achieve your weight gain goals. Adjust your workout plan as needed to continue making progress.

9. Listen to Your Body: Pay attention to how your body responds to exercise. If you feel overly fatigued or are experiencing difficulty gaining weight, consider adjusting your workout routine or seeking guidance from a certified fitness trainer or healthcare professional.

10. Consider High-Intensity Interval Training (HIIT): If you prefer more intense cardiovascular workouts, consider incorporating short bursts of high-intensity interval training (HIIT). HIIT can be effective for cardiovascular fitness while minimizing the overall time spent on cardio.

Remember, the primary focus for weight gain should be on resistance training and providing your body with enough calories and nutrients to support muscle growth. Cardiovascular exercise can complement your routine and contribute to overall fitness and well-being, but it should be balanced appropriately to prevent excessive calorie expenditure that may hinder weight gain efforts.

Chapter 5: Overcoming Weight Gain Challenges

Weight gain, like any health journey, can present its own set of challenges. However, with determination and the right strategies, you can overcome these obstacles and continue progressing towards your goals. In this chapter, we will explore some common challenges associated with weight gain and discuss effective ways to overcome them.

• • • •

Dealing with Weight Gain Plateaus:

Weight gain plateaus can be disheartening, but it's important to remember that they are a natural part of the process. As you gain weight and build muscle, your body adapts to the changes, and the rate of weight gain may slow down temporarily. Here are some strategies to deal with weight gain plateaus:

A. Stay Consistent: Plateaus can test your patience, but it's crucial to stay consistent with your healthy eating and exercise habits. Even though the scale may not show progress, your body is likely still benefiting from the lifestyle changes you've made.

b. Reevaluate Your Plan: Take a closer look at your diet and exercise routine. Consider tracking your food intake and activity levels to ensure you are maintaining a calorie surplus. You may need to adjust your caloric intake or mix up your workouts to challenge your body and break through the plateau.

c. Monitor Non-Scale Progress: While the scale may not be moving, focus on the non-scale victories you've achieved. Celebrate improvements in strength, endurance, flexibility, and overall well-being. Recognizing these positive changes can keep you motivated during plateaus.

Staying Motivated and Focused on Your Goals:

Maintaining motivation throughout your weight gain journey can be challenging, especially when progress seems slow. Here are some strategies to help you stay motivated and focused:

a. Set Short-Term Goals: Break your long-term weight gain goal into smaller, manageable milestones. Celebrate each achievement along the way. These short-term goals provide a sense of accomplishment and keep you motivated for the long run.

b. Visualize Success: Take a few moments each day to visualize yourself reaching your weight gain goals. Imagine how you will feel, look, and the positive impact on your life. Visualization can reinforce your commitment to success.

c. Find Support: Seek out support from friends, family, or join a weight gain support group. Surrounding yourself with like-minded individuals can provide encouragement, accountability, and a sense of community during your journey.

Strategies to Overcome Common Obstacles:

Weight gain can present various obstacles that may hinder your progress. Here are some effective strategies to overcome these challenges:

A. Time Management: Time constraints can make it challenging to prioritize healthy eating and exercise. Plan your meals and workouts in advance, and find time-saving strategies, such as meal prepping and quick, effective workouts.

b. Mindful Eating: Emotional eating can be a stumbling block for weight gain. Practice mindful eating by paying attention to hunger cues, eating slowly, and savoring your food. Avoid using food as a coping mechanism for stress or emotions.

c. Travel and Social Events: Traveling and social gatherings can disrupt your routine, making it challenging to stick to your weight gain plan. Plan ahead by researching healthier food options, packing snacks, and finding opportunities for physical activity during your trips.

Managing Social and Emotional Aspects of Weight Gain:

Weight gain can trigger various emotions and affect your social interactions. Here's how to handle these aspects:

A. Communicate with Loved Ones: Share your weight gain journey with friends and family. Explain your goals and the reasons behind your lifestyle changes. Seek understanding and support from those close to you.

b. Address Emotional Eating: Emotional eating can be a coping mechanism for stress, boredom, or sadness. Find alternative ways to deal with emotions, such as going for a walk, meditating, journaling, or engaging in a hobby.

c. Embrace Body Positivity: Weight gain may come with body image concerns. Focus on the positive changes you're making for your health and well-being, rather than solely focusing on the number on the scale. Embrace body positivity and practice self-acceptance.

By implementing these strategies and maintaining a positive mindset, you can overcome obstacles and stay on track with your weight gain goals. Remember that setbacks are normal, and the journey to a healthier lifestyle is a gradual process. Celebrate your successes, learn from challenges, and keep moving forward with determination and resilience.

Chapter 6: Maintaining Your Weight Gain

Maintaining your weight gain is just as important as achieving it. After putting in the effort to gain weight, it's essential to sustain your progress and ensure that you continue to support your body's needs. Here are some tips to help you maintain your weight gain:

1. Continue Strength Training: Keep up with your regular strength training routine to maintain the muscle mass you've gained. Consistent resistance training is crucial for preventing muscle loss and keeping your metabolism active.

2. Adjust Caloric Intake: As your weight increases, your caloric needs may change. Reevaluate your calorie intake and adjust it accordingly to match your current weight and activity level. Aim for a balance between the calories you consume and the energy you expend to maintain your weight.

3. Eat a Balanced Diet: Continue to focus on a balanced diet that includes a variety of nutrient-dense foods. Include plenty of fruits, vegetables, whole grains, lean proteins, and healthy fats to support your overall health and well-being.

4. Protein Intake: Protein is essential for maintaining muscle mass. Be sure to consume an adequate amount of protein in your diet to support muscle repair and recovery.

5. Monitor Your Progress: Regularly track your weight and body measurements to ensure you're maintaining your weight gain. This will help you identify any fluctuations or changes that may require adjustments to your diet or exercise routine.

6. Avoid Crash Diets: Avoid drastic changes to your diet or engaging in crash diets to lose weight quickly. Such approaches can lead to muscle loss and other health issues. Instead, focus on maintaining a healthy and sustainable eating pattern.

7. Stay Active: Even if you've achieved your weight gain goals,

don't become sedentary. Stay active and engage in regular physical activity to maintain your fitness level and overall health.

8. Get Enough Sleep: Adequate sleep is crucial for your body's recovery and overall well-being. Aim for 7-9 hours of quality sleep each night to support your weight maintenance efforts.

9. Manage Stress: High levels of stress can affect your eating habits and may lead to unhealthy behaviors. Find healthy ways to manage stress, such as through exercise, meditation, or hobbies you enjoy.

10. Seek Support: Surround yourself with supportive friends, family, or a support group to help you stay motivated and accountable in maintaining your weight gain.

Remember that maintaining weight gain is an ongoing process that requires consistent effort and a healthy lifestyle. Embrace the positive changes you've made and continue to prioritize your physical and mental well-being. If you have any concerns or specific health goals, consider seeking guidance from a registered dietitian or a healthcare professional to ensure that you're on the right track and maintaining your weight gain in a healthy way.

Creating a sustainable and healthy lifestyle

Creating a sustainable and healthy lifestyle is crucial for maintaining weight gain in a way that supports overall well-being. When you adopt a balanced approach to nutrition, exercise, and self-care, you can sustain your weight gain efforts and avoid the common pitfalls of yo-yo dieting. Here's how a sustainable and healthy lifestyle can help you maintain weight gain:

1. Balanced Nutrition: A sustainable and healthy lifestyle focuses on a balanced diet that includes a variety of nutrient-dense

foods. By nourishing your body with the right nutrients, you support muscle maintenance and overall health.

2. Portion Control: Practicing portion control helps you manage your calorie intake and avoid overeating, which can lead to unwanted weight gain. Being mindful of portion sizes allows you to enjoy your favorite foods while still maintaining a healthy balance.

3. Regular Exercise: Incorporating regular physical activity into your lifestyle, such as strength training and cardiovascular workouts, helps maintain muscle mass and supports a healthy metabolism. Exercise also enhances your overall fitness and well-being.

4. Building Healthy Habits: By creating sustainable habits around nutrition and exercise, you're more likely to stick with them in the long run. Consistency is key to maintaining weight gain and overall health.

5. Mindful Eating: Practicing mindful eating encourages you to be present during meals, pay attention to hunger cues, and make conscious food choices. This helps prevent mindless snacking or emotional eating, which can lead to weight fluctuations.

6. Adequate Sleep: Prioritizing quality sleep is essential for hormone regulation and overall health. Lack of sleep can disrupt hunger hormones and lead to weight gain, so ensuring sufficient rest supports your weight maintenance efforts.

7. Stress Management: Managing stress through various techniques like meditation, yoga, or spending time in nature can prevent emotional eating and support a healthy relationship with food.

8. Balanced Approach: Avoid extreme diets or restrictive eating patterns, as they are difficult to maintain and often lead to rebound weight gain. Embrace a balanced approach to nutrition that allows for flexibility and enjoyment.

9. Self-Compassion: Be kind to yourself and avoid harsh self-criticism. Weight maintenance is a journey, and setbacks may occur. Practice self-compassion and focus on progress rather than perfection.

10. Seek Support: Surround yourself with a supportive network of friends, family, or support groups who understand your goals and can provide encouragement. Having a support system can help you stay motivated and accountable.

11. Flexibility and Adaptability: Embrace flexibility in your lifestyle, as life may present unexpected challenges or changes. Be willing to adapt your nutrition and exercise routine as needed to accommodate different situations.

By creating a sustainable and healthy lifestyle, you build a foundation for lasting weight maintenance and overall well-being. When you approach weight gain and maintenance with a holistic mindset, it becomes a natural part of your life rather than a temporary endeavor. Remember that healthy living is a lifelong journey, and the choices you make today will impact your well-being in the long term.

Celebrating your weight gain success

Celebrating your weight gain success is a great way to acknowledge your hard work, boost your motivation, and reinforce positive habits. Here are five effective ways to celebrate your weight gain success:

1. Personal Rewards: Treat yourself to a personal reward that aligns with your interests and values. It could be buying a new outfit that makes you feel confident and comfortable in your body, investing in a fitness-related gadget or equipment, or indulging in a relaxing self-care activity like a massage or spa day.

2. Social Celebration: Share your success with friends and family

by hosting a small gathering or dinner. This not only allows you to celebrate your achievement but also fosters a supportive environment that encourages you to maintain your healthy habits.

3. Progress Photos: Take progress photos and create a visual timeline of your weight gain journey. Seeing the changes in your body over time can be incredibly motivating and serves as a reminder of your accomplishments.

4. Set New Fitness Goals: Celebrate by setting new fitness or health-related goals that challenge you to continue improving. Whether it's increasing the weight you can lift, achieving a fitness milestone, or signing up for a physical event like a charity run or a fitness challenge, having a new goal can keep you focused and excited.

5. Reflect and Express Gratitude: Take time to reflect on your weight gain journey and express gratitude for the progress you've made. Write in a journal about the positive changes you've experienced, the lessons you've learned, and the reasons you are proud of yourself. Practicing gratitude can boost your overall well-being and reinforce a positive mindset.

Remember that celebrating your weight gain success should be a personal and meaningful experience. Avoid comparing your achievements to others and focus on your unique journey and progress. Celebrate your accomplishments in a way that aligns with your values and reinforces your commitment to a healthy and sustainable lifestyle. Celebrating your success can help you maintain your weight gain efforts and continue making positive choices for your overall well-being.

Conclusion

In conclusion, celebrating your weight gain success is an important aspect of maintaining a healthy and sustainable lifestyle. Achieving weight gain requires dedication, hard work, and perseverance, and acknowledging your progress is vital for staying motivated and committed to your goals.

By celebrating your weight gain success, you reinforce positive habits and behaviors, boost your self-confidence, and foster a positive mindset. It's essential to focus on non-scale victories, such as increased energy, improved strength, and enhanced overall well-being, as these achievements are equally valuable as the numbers on the scale.

Remember that weight gain is a journey, and it's normal to face challenges along the way. Be kind to yourself and practice self-compassion, celebrating both small and significant milestones. Setting new goals and maintaining a supportive environment can help you sustain your achievements and continue thriving in your pursuit of a balanced and fulfilling life.

Embrace a sustainable and healthy lifestyle that prioritizes balanced nutrition, regular exercise, adequate rest, and stress management. By creating a positive and nurturing environment for yourself, you set the foundation for long-term success in maintaining your weight gain and overall well-being.

Ultimately, celebrating your weight gain success is not just about reaching a specific number on the scale; it's about embracing the journey of self-improvement, self-care, and personal growth. Cherish the progress you've made, and use each success as motivation to continue moving forward on your path to a healthier and happier you.